ALICIA NGIAM

BSc. Psych., UIU; MEd. Guidance and Counseling, UPM, CCHO, Clarity Group

PERMA+

THE SCIENCE OF FLOURISHING

A Quick Guide to Self-Transformation | Awaken Your Potential

www.PositivePsychologyPractice.org

ALICIA NGIAM

BSc. Psych., UIU; MEd. Guidance and Counseling, UPM, CCHO, Clarity Group

PERMA+

THE SCIENCE OF FLOURISHING

A Quick Guide to Self-Transformation |
Awaken Your Potential

www.PositivePsychologyPractice.org

PERMA+: The Science of Flourishing

Copyright © 2022 Alicia Ngiam

All Rights Reserved

Disclaimer

Every care has been taken to ensure that the knowledge and techniques in this book are workable and safe. Success using this knowledge and model varies from person to person. This booklet as a guide is very helpful, but should not be used as a total substitute for consultation with a mental health professional.

First Printing: August 2022
ISBN: 9798354107575

About the Author

Alicia Ngiam *(Bsc. Psy., UIU, MEd. Guidance and Counseling, UPM, CCHO, Clariti Group)*

Alicia Ngiam (BSc. Psy., UIU, MEd. Guidance and Counseling, UPM - in progress) was awarded the Certified Chief Happiness Officer title in 2020, in the midst of lockdowns of the coronavirus pandemic, making her the first in Malaysia to receive such title for her works. Alicia has spent the past 8 years studying and researching about trauma recovery, brain plasticity, resilience, and positive psychology. In 2016 she became the first undergraduate student on-campus to conduct a quasi-experimental research on light and psychological functions in humans. This research was later published in Germany. She has also worked with trauma survivors and PTSD. Her services can be found on PositivePsychologyPractice.org and she is also the founder of Happiness Malaysia, an initiative to increase happiness in Malaysia. She also manages an online activity booking platform for adventures and retreats in Malaysia.

Foreword

In a world tainted with trauma, pain, and suffering, it is becoming increasingly inevitable that these are matters that we have to live with. Yet despite all odds, there are countless people who manage to "make it" and achieve whatever they have ever dreamed of.

This book will help you:
- Gain more confidence
- Increase your self-esteem
- Reduce depression, anxiety, and shame
- Reduce and eliminate PTSD
- Decrease psychosomatic illness
- Achieve work-life balance
- Achieve meaning
- Enhance relationships
- Improve sleep hygiene
- Increase sales and workplace productivity
- And most of all, increase overall happiness!

The FIVE PLUS principles of positive psychology serve as pillars of subjective well-being that everyone can follow, regardless of age, gender, and race. My hope is that I have written this book in the simplest terms so that it is easy to understand.

PERMA+: An Overview

Resilience: Defined as the ability to bounce back after adversity.

For several centuries, resilience was thought to be a unique gift. Today, however, we know that resilience is a characteristic that can be learned. The science of resilience focuses on building strengths, and PERMA+ helps you achieve just that. This booklet will help you become more resilient, a much-needed trait of the 21st century, through a basic overview of PERMA+.

The pillars of positive Psychology are Positive Emotions, Engagement, Relationships, Meaning, and Achievement, PLUS Optimism, Exercise, Sleep, and Nutrition. These are the factors that contribute to overall subjective well-being, and when combined together, builds and individual's resilience and allows flourishing to one's potential.

Contrary to psychology in the past which focused solely on history and negative experiences and thoughts, positive psychology looks beyond that and highlights the future and positive experiences. PERMA+ serves as fundamental building blocks in the process of constructing a stronger, happier well-being. This turn in mental health was put forward by Dr Martin Seligman, who is one of the founding fathers of positive psychology, in the year 1998, when he was elected President of the American Psychological Association. PERMA+ has since been the focus of positive psychology, and it has been broken down further to deepen the understanding of the framework. Positive psychology is a combination of philosophy and psychology in one package. The shift of focus from one's history to examining strengths is a leap in the field that is going beyond boundaries.

Positive psychology looks beyond past experiences and present events in an individual's life as guidance towards a life of flourishing. Negative and positive experiences are both accountable in building up personality and choices in life. In addition, positive psychology follows a 360-degree framework.

By a 360-degree framework, this means that optimum well-being is achieved via both physical and mental health. This is a huge turning point in psychology as older schools of psychology solely focused on mental health. Present-day researchers consider the influence of physical health on mental well-being, and vice versa - therefore it is necessary to consider both factors at once when administering treatment.

The elements of PERMA+ work together to enhance resilience and subjective well-being. This increases the threshold to face adversities, and helps bring people and communities stand back on their feet again to recover and run and play again.

The Benefits of Resilience:

- Emotional stability
- Increased capacity to overcome adversities
- Learned hopefulness
- Better coping strategies
- Higher tolerance threshold for events that may otherwise be traumatic
- Decreased likelihood of psychosis
- Decreased episodes of depression
- Higher subjective well-being
- Matured form of happiness
- Peak productivity
- Optimized workplace performance
- Improves relationships and marriages

With resilience as the main contributing factor in cultivating happiness, expanding the capacity to bounce back from hardships has definitely gained importance in the field of positive psychology. In addition, research has now shown that resilience is a characteristic that can be learned and improved through practice. Utilizing PERMA+ principles that have been listed out in this book as a guide can help promote resilience, therefore reinforcing marriages, families, teams, and work culture.

Positive Emotions

MORE THAN JUST HAPPY

Positive emotions encompass much more than just happiness. As the first component of PERMA+, positive emotion encompass joy, love, success, grace, patience, and hope, including others. 26 positive emotions have been listed down altogether, that being as follows:

- joy
- gratitude
- serenity
- interest
- hope
- pride
- amusement
- happiness
- inspiration
- awe
- elevation
- altruism
- satisfaction
- relief
- affection
- optimism
- cheerfulness
- surprise
- confidence
- respect
- enthusiasm
- euphoria

It is not necessary to experience all of these emotions at once. However, experiencing a build-up of various positive emotions leads to flourishing. The ability to experience such emotions is partly due also to our genetic predisposition. In addition, positive emotions reduce the likelihood of diseases, such as myocarditis and heart failure, as well as increase the speed of recovery from illnesses. Working on positive emotions enhances coping mechanisms and helps one deal with stressors. Experiencing positive emotions also boosts one's adaptability to major life changes.

Engagement

When one is engaged, it means that one is so involved in an activity that he or she loses track of time and energy. The adage, "Time flies when you are having fun", is very relatable to the second component of PERMA+. According to Dr Mihalyi Csikzentmihalyi (1940 - 2021) who discovered flow theory, one experiences engagement when involved in a challenging activity that is in line with our strengths. And when that occurs, one achieves what is known as the state of flow. This way, one is able to hone his strengths. There are 220 character strengths identified to date, all of them, including virtue, reliability, and honesty contribute to an improved well-being. Constantly being engaged and in the state of flow also increases work productivity and peak performances. To do this, reflect on what you find interesting to do. How do you like to spend your free time? It is also a great idea to have many interests so that we can shift from one to another whenever the need arises.

Relationships

BEYOND HUMAN CONNECTIONS

Humans are social creatures, regardless whether a person is an introvert or an extrovert. Human connection at an interpersonal, social, communal, and familial level play a huge role in optimal well-being. Relationships that cultivate meaning create a positive impact on resilience construction also. Being able to access support, having supportive family, and supportive friends increases morale. As the saying goes, it takes a village to raise a child. The quality of relationships have an effect on one's well-being, and therefore when seeking friendships it is encouraged to look for quality rather than quantity.

Getting in touch with a long-lost friend or family member rekindles connections and feelings of satisfaction and gratefulness, whereas creating new ones promotes a sense of belonging and inclusion.

Meaning

LIVING A PURPOSE-DRIVEN LIFE

Having a positive outlook in life does not mean one will not encounter adverse events. To face challenges that life throws from time to time requires one to be realistic. Suffering makes up a huge part of life, and as soon as one realizes that, the higher his subjective well-being will be. Developing meaning helps one cultivate ikigai, the reason for being (which will be discussed more on PositivePsychologyPractice.org). Greek philosopher Socrates once said: "The unexamined life is not worth living." Life is a unique blend of positives and negatives; it is the way these experiences are handled that create a positive outcome. Gain a deeper insight, a more in-depth understanding of circumstances that revolve around you. Face adversities with matured happiness.

To learn more about meaning and ikigai check out PositivePsychologyPractice.org.

Achievement

According to Abraham Maslow's Heirarchy of Needs, self-actualization significantly increases self-worth and value. Self-actualization is realized when one has reached the peak of life and career where everything is running smoothly. Having accomplished our goals leaves us with a sense of achievement. This greatly contributes to our well-being and improves our self-esteem and confidence. Yet, why are a majority of people still left feeling unsatisfied, angry, and unhappy?

Obviously, other factors are at play, one of which is meaning. Deriving meaning from life's work gives us a sense of purpose, something to live for despite the inevitable challenges and suffering of today's world. Researchers and psychologists have long observed the lives of the Japanese, who work a huge part of their lives and are very stringent about protocol, yet live to ripe old age. What must be their secret?

Much of what we know about meaning today has been long been taught in Japan. Its nature-oriented culture is filled with reconnection with ancestors, with trees, with birds, the oceans - and even stones. It is not a surprise, then, for psychologists to have the urge to understand more about Japan's unique culture. What they found is that the people of the land of the rising sunlive by the concept of *ikigai*; having a reason to live, to exist, and to flourish.

It is, as these researchers have observed, the very reason why certain few have successfully managed to do well despite the many challenges that come their way.

Optimism

A POSITIVE OUTLOOK

Positive psychology is the science of contructing resilience, with flourishing as the ultimate goal. That is, in the aftermath of suffering, one seeks to not only heal but also to go beyond that and experience self-transcendence, attaining ikigai. Optimism plays an important role in learning to construct resilience by maintaining a positive outlook on the ups and downs of life. People who are optimistic are less stressful in adverse circumstances and tend to have longer lasting relationships, be it personal or work. People who have a sense of humor tend to experience speedier recovery from setbacks. To be realistically optimistic, make small, bite-sized goals that are easier to reach.

Nutrition

MINDFULNESS WITH WHAT WE EAT

Nearly everything we eat today consists of processed foods, which have high sodium, fat, and cholesterol content. These substances can be potentially harmful to our health. Artherosclerosis, high blood pressure, diabetes, and myocarditis are just a few illnesses of the body that are lethal if left untreated. Our culture is struggling with maintaining the "perfect" body image; skinny models flaunt the media while food chains promote a never-ending array of fat-laden foods. Since whatever we eat circulates all around the body including the brain via the bloodstream, we must be mindful of what we eat on a daily basis and realize that this has an impact on our well-being.

MINDFULNESS WITH WHAT WE EAT

Sleep

MORE THAN A GOOD NIGHT

Sleep is extremely vital to our well-being. Much of mental illness today is due to the very lack of sleep. During sleep, the body has the opportunity to repair itself; to replenish cells and nutrients to damaged tissues; to detoxify blood; and the mind to rest and reflect. In 2016, I conducted a quasi-experimental research on the effects of the lack of light on psychological functions, especially sleep and mood. Though it may sound mundane, the research to this day is being sought after by thousands of researchers all around the world. I had my participants stay in a room with no light for a few hours and recorded their thoughts and feelings. Every individual's sleep is actually regulated by the CLOCK gene which is found in the suprachiasmatic nucleus (SCN) in the brain. What does this CLOCK gene do? As the name suggests, this special gene determines how and when and how much sleep one is going to have, in what we call the circardian rhythm, or body clock. The CLOCK gene, together with the synthesis of serotonin, establishes the body's sleep homeostasis. Genes may take a longer time to alter, but we can definitely manipulate serotonin levels in our blood through the foods we eat, as well as our environment. The SCN responds to serotonin levels and CLOCK gene expression; serotonin on the other hand is induced during darkness. Therefore we can work around adjusting how much light we expose ourselves to on a daily basis. The average amount of sleep for an adult is 7-9 hours; for children it is 10 hours.

Things that we can do to improve sleep:
- Reduce TV time
- Switch off mobile/digital devices during bedtime
- Keep a strict sleep schedule
- Drink warm milk
- Listen to ASMR
- Re-make a comfortable bed
- Connect with Nature during the day
- Make sure bedroom is completely dark
- Use an eye mask/ear buds while sleeping
- Take hot baths to soothe the nervous system
- Schedule a spa day, or give yourself a bath scrub once every week

For more information look up Light Deprivation and Its Effects (Ngiam, 2016). If you would like to work on your sleep hygiene, book your consultation on PositivePsychologyPractice.org.

EXERCISE

MOVING AWAY FROM SEDENTARY LIFESTYLES

A great way to increase neurogenesis, or growth of neurons in the brain, is by becoming physically active. Through regular exercise, dopamine, the happiness chemical - along with other neurotransmitters - is increased, which contributes to happiness. Exercise promotes neuroplasticity, by bringing more oxygen to the brain thus allowing the brain cells to grow and proliferate. Not only that, exercise improves blood circulation. Being consistent makes you more disciplined, improves sleep, gets your metabolic functions working smoothly, and increases resilience. Over time, you start to see the results: A toned body, firmer muscles, weight loss, etc. When you exercise, your body produces adenosine triphosphate, or ATP, which is really a form of energy. This explains why we feel hot and sweaty during exercise. Now, here's the thing: The longer we spend doing a particular exercise at any one time, the more our muscles produce what is known as lactic acid. This is the substance that gives our muscles a sore feeling. You definitely have heard of fitness enthusiasts saying, "No pain, no gain." Exercise takes into effect when you get past that soreness produced by the lactic acid in your muscles. In addition, oxygen intake will increase, replenishing cells in the entire body with oxygen.

It has been mentioned that exercise promotes resilience. By definition, resilience simply means bouncing back in the face of adversity. Exercise helps us grow mentally and prepare us psychologically to face challenges, something that is getting more and more of a necessity in a more-than-ever rapidly changing world. You can learn more about resilience on my website PositivePsychologyPractice.org.

List of Values

Acceptance
Achievement
Advancement
Adventure
Affection
Altruism
Arts
Awareness
Beauty
Bravery
Challenge
Change
Community
Compassion
Competence
Competition
Completion
Connectedness
Cooperation
Collaboration
Country
Creativity
Decisiveness
Democracy
Design
Discovery
Diversity
Environmental
Awareness

Education
Economic
Security
Effectiveness
Efficiency
Elegance
Entertainment
Enlightenment
Equality
Ethics
Excellence
Excitement
Experiment
Expertise
Exhilaration
Fairness
Fame
Family
Happiness
Fast Pace
Freedom
Friendship
Fun
Grace
Growth
Harmony
Health
Helping Others
Helping Society

Honesty
Humor
Imagination
Independence
Improvement
Influencing Others
Inner Harmony
Inspiration
Integrity
Intellect
Involvement
Knowledge
Leadership
Learning
Loyalty
Magnificence
Making a Difference
Mastery
Meaningful Work
Money
Morality
Mystery
Nature
Openness
Originality
Order
Passion
Peace
Personal Development

Personal Expression
Ministering
Money
Morality
Mystery
Nature
Openness
Originality
Order
Passion
Peace
Personal Development
Personal Expression
Planning
Play
Pleasure
Power
Privacy
Purity
Quality
Reassurance
Recognition
Relationships
Religion
Reputation
Responsibility
Risk Safety
Self Respect
Sensibility

Service
Sexuality
Sophistication
Spark
Speculation
Spirituality
Stability
Status
Success
Teaching
Tenderness
Thrill
Unity
Variety
Wealth
Winning
Wisdom

FREE TOOL: IDENTIFYING VALUES

Building resilience starts from our values, which provides us the strength that we need. Take some time to reflect on a life changing event that you have experienced. Find a little quiet corner where you can sit comfortably and think. What value do you identify with?

1. Describe a life-changing event.

-

2. Identify reasons to go through the event.

3. Identify the values that you upheld in order to pull
   through.

4. Look for ways to stay in touch with your values.
   Your values are what make you unique and stand out
   from the rest of the crowd.

SALES CHANNEL

Camps and workshops on happiness and positive psychology are available throughout the year.

Happiness Retreats
Resilience Masterclass
Annual Memberships
Consulting Packages
Merchandise

Book on positivepsychologypractice.org or drop an email to positivepsychologypractice@gmail.com today!!

Follow us on social media:

Positive Psychology Practice

@positivepsychologypractice

Happiness Malaysia

@happinessmalaysia

REFERENCES

Alberts, H., Wells, L., Latif, S., Nash, J., Sutton, J., & Schaffner, A. K. (2020). Positivepsychology.com.

Ngiam, A. (2016). Light deprivation and its effects, Lambert Publishing. shorturl.at/anpW9.

Ngiam, A. (2021). Positivepsychologypractice.org.

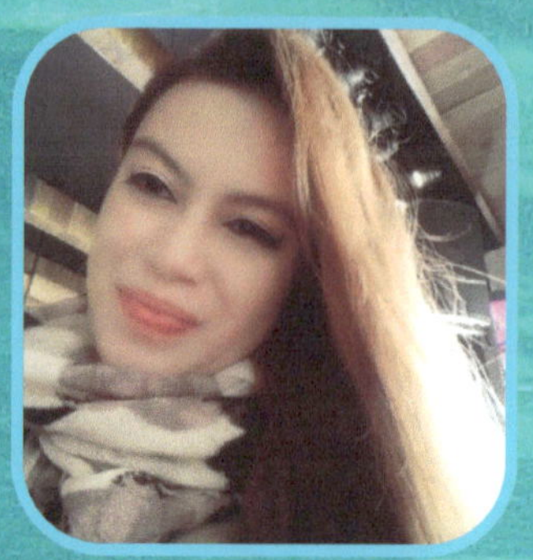

Alicia Ngiam is an author and the founder of PositivePsychologyPractic.org and TRIPPI. She has managed teams and hosted projects related to positive psychology. She has also started the Happiness Malaysia initiative, and is currently pursuing her Masters of Education in Guidance and Counseling in Universiti Putra Malaysia.

"The short e-book is clear, concise and packed full of information. HUGE congratulations for making this happen. You are bringing so much joy to the world and it's an honour to know you." - **Belinda Jane Dolan (CEO, World Happiness Project)**

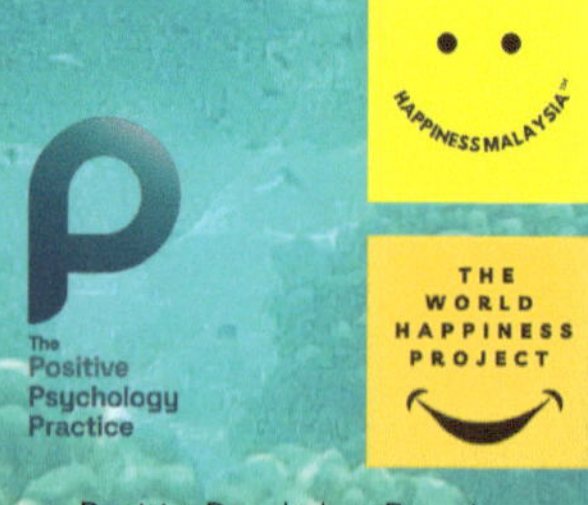

www.PositivePsychologyPractice.org

www.ingramcontent.com/pod-product-compliance
Lightning Source LLC
Chambersburg PA
CBHW040252240726
48664CB00001B/369